ANYA GORE was born in London, and has a German/
Russian background. In her early twenties she lived in
Florence, Italy, for three years, working in publishing
and co-founding an English-speaking theatre.

On returning to England, she trained in drama at
the Bristol Old Vic Theatre School and did a variety of
professional work. During this time, she became
interested in massage, reflexology and a holistic
approach to good health. She now works as a full-time
trained reflexologist and masseuse.

ALTERNATIVE HEALTH

REFLEXOLOGY

ANYA GORE

ILLUSTRATED BY SHAUN WILLIAMS

An OPTIMA book

© Anya Gore, 1990

First published in 1990 by
Macdonald Optima, a division of
Macdonald & Co. (Publishers) Ltd

A member of Maxwell Macmillan Pergamon Publishing Corporation

All rights reserved

British Library Cataloguing in Publication Data

Gore, Anya
    Reflexology.
    1. Man. Therapy. Use of reflex massage of hands and feet
    I. Title   II. Series
    615.8'22

    ISBN 0-356-17180-9

Macdonald & Co. (Publishers) Ltd
Orbit House
1 New Fetter Lane
London EC4A 1AR

Photoset in Century Schoolbook by
𝍓 Tek Art Ltd, Croydon, Surrey

Printed and bound in Great Britain by
The Guernsey Press

DEDICATION

For Nick West, with all my love.

CONTENTS

ACKNOWLEDGMENTS

My grateful thanks to Peter Gore for his help with the word processor. Special thanks to Nick West for his invaluable, patient and perceptive help in reading the manuscript and in discussing ideas with me. And my thanks to everyone who has helped me on my way, and thereby contributed to this book.

INTRODUCTION

This book is designed to give a comprehensive overview
of what reflexology is, how it is thought to work, what
it feels like to experience it, and what it can do for you.
I have attempted to discuss all of this within a wider
framework which expresses a philosophy of the nature
of health and disease and an approach to life which
makes sense to me.

The book has been written from the standpoint of my
own experience of reflexology, both as a practitioner
and as a patient. It therefore provides a practical guide
to the subject, and will, I hope, make it more
accessible. Reflexology is one of the oldest known
methods of natural healing, and was used by several
ancient civilizations, but our modern understanding of
the complexities of the physical body can only serve to
enhance the quality of the treatments. Reflexology is a
simple yet effective system of foot (and hand) massage
and manipulation, the effects of which not only are felt
all over the body, but also benefit the person's
emotional and mental state.

At various points in the book, I refer to the different
'levels' of our being. To explain briefly, these can be
seen as the physical, mental, emotional and
imaginative levels. We are probably most familiar with
the physical level, because we can see and feel our
bodies. The mental level at which we exist is also very
much a conscious level – the level of thinking, logic,
often of 'churning' ideas around in our heads. If we are

too focused on this level, it can cause us discomfort, and at times we may feel we are 'going round in circles'. The emotional level, which is sometimes further from our conscious reach, is none the less just as real. At times we are of course very aware of our emotions – and, as will be seen, they have a profound effect also on our minds and bodies. When we get out of touch with our emotions, a physical symptom can occur to remind us to 'tune in'. The imaginative/creative level of our being is sometimes even more blocked off from our everyday awareness. We could also term this the spiritual level (and by using that word I am not subscribing to any particular belief system) – and this is of course just as important as the other levels.

In fact all these levels are integral to who we are, and they all interact and affect each other. The four broad categories mentioned do, however, provide a good basis from which to look at ourselves and one another. Reflexology can help open up awareness to the existence and interplay of all these levels, and therefore to many aspects of our being, and can help us towards a true feeling of satisfaction.

Quite simply, the state of relaxation brought about through reflexology, together with the specific effects of deeper manipulation of the reflex points, encourages the patient towards a happier and stronger experience of life. This book helps to explain how this may be achieved.

I hope that this book will remove any apprehension that may be felt about trying an unfamiliar therapy, and it is with this in mind that I have included a chapter on the self-treatment of some common complaints, although clearly there is no real substitute for treatments by a professional reflexologist. It is worth mentioning that you do not actually need to be ill to benefit from reflexology treatment. People in generally good health can also be helped because reflexology is in addition a preventative therapy, and because it is deeply relaxing.

Reflexology's ancient origins in a sense add to the mystery of how it actually works, and yet the fact that it is still (and these days increasingly) practised shows that it is a very valid system of healing, and one which works. It may be that when it originated explanations existed, even perhaps so-called 'scientific' ones, and that we have lost access to that way of analysing how the treatment works. It seems, though, that there is no adequate scientific explanation at present for how reflexology works, so all we can do is see and experience the results.

It is hoped that by the end of this book you will have gained further insight into the whole area of your health, and that you will be able to see yourself and your ability to be responsible for your life and well-being in a new and positive way.

1
WHAT IS REFLEXOLOGY?

A BRIEF HISTORY

Reflexology is an ancient healing art using pressure,
especially on certain points on the feet. It is a
technique which goes back thousands of years. The
Chinese practised a form of pressure therapy which is
thought to have developed alongside acupuncture as
long ago as 3000 BC. It was certainly practised in
Ancient Egypt in 2330 BC, as paintings on the
Physician's Tomb in Saqqara illustrate.

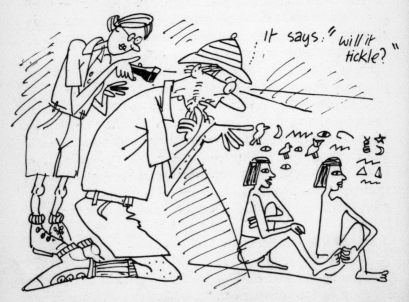

It says: "will it tickle?"

REFLEXOLOGY WAS PRACTISED IN ANCIENT EGYPT

Little is known about the development of reflexology since these ancient times. There seems to be no real documentation or historical evidence of it again until the publication of several books on the subject in Europe in the sixteenth century, for instance by the physicians Adamus and A'tatis in 1582, and by a Dr Bell in Leipzig. We must assume, however, that the skill continued to be passed down in some way in the interim.

It was not until early this century, however, that real interest in the subject was created in the West. In 1913 an American ear, nose and throat specialist, Dr William H. Fitzgerald, started researching into this method of healing, later to be called 'zone therapy'. He had worked for two years in Vienna, where he probably first came across the subject, and on returning to America he developed his work further and started to apply it, initially amidst much scepticism.

Fitzgerald divided the body into ten vertical zones, five on each side of the body (see the diagram on page 6). He found that there was an energy link between all parts of the body falling within a particular zone, and that by applying pressure to one area, pain could be reduced in other areas within that zone.

Fitzgerald employed different instruments to apply pressure, mainly to the fingers and hands. He used clothes pegs over the finger tips, combs held tightly by the hands, and elastic bands around the fingers. These were the usual methods, but pressure was sometimes similarly applied to the toes, ankles, wrists, elbows and knees. After much experimentation, it became clear that pressure applied to the ends of a finger or corresponding toe could affect all areas within that zone.

Fitzgerald also identified ten zones on the tongue, five on each side of a middle line, and divided the soft palate into ten zones, though of course these areas are sometimes inconvenient to treat. Reflexes for the whole body can also be found in the ears, but again these are

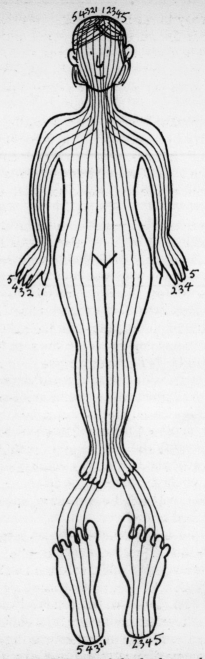

The ten vertical zones of the body, and how they correspond to the soles of the feet.

not very easy to reach precisely with the fingers. He noted particular success in treating ailments such as headaches, eye conditions, goitres, fibroids in the womb, breast lumps and breathing problems. Of his cases, 65 to 75 per cent were successfully treated – a high rate.

The term 'zone therapy' was actually coined early this century by a colleague and student of Fitzgerald's, Dr Edwin F. Bowers, who was a medical critic and writer from New York. Other contributors to the development of the technique were three American doctors, George Starr White, Joe Riley and Elizabeth Riley. Joe Riley introduced something called 'hook work', a technique whereby the practitioner hooked their hands over a part of the body in order to manipulate tissue or joints, and he related this closely to the zone system, for instance treating the elbow to affect the knee (see the figure on page 13).

Eunice D. Ingham, a pupil of Joe Riley, was the real founder of reflexology as we know it in the West today. She developed the Ingham compression method of reflexology, and her books, *Stories the Feet Can Tell* and *Stories the Feet Have Told*, are classics on the subject. The Ingham method concentrated on reflexes found on the soles and tops of the feet and the toes. Through experimentation, and by noting the consistency of the results, she managed to project the various parts of the body on to specific areas of the feet, and so perfected the technique of reflexology as it is currently practised.

One of Ingham's students, Doreen Bayly, was largely responsible for the introduction of reflexology to Britain in the early 1960s, starting a school of reflexology and running a successful practice. At first there was little interest, but gradually, largely due to Bayly's work, enthusiasm for the technique spread. In recent years, with the ever accelerating interest in, and need for, alternative approaches to health, reflexology has become more and more popular. It is one of the

most effective alternative therapies, a fact often belied
by its simplicity, because there is a tendency for simple
techniques to be considered less effective than
complicated ones. In fact the reverse is sometimes true.
A technique like reflexology is popular not only
because of its remarkable efficacy, but because it is
uncomplicated for the recipient – all you have to do is
take your shoes and socks off and lie down! It can also
feel delightful to have your feet manipulated.

THE ZONES OF THE BODY

As already mentioned, Fitzgerald and his colleagues
realized that the body could be divided into ten
longitudinal zones, extending throughout the body,
with five zones on each side of a medial line. An organ
existing in a specific zone of the body will have its
reflex point in the same zone of the foot. For example,
the left kidney, found in zones two and three of the
body, has its reflex point in zones two and three of the
left foot. As the diagram opposite shows, the ten zones
are equal in width, and go through the body from front
to back, dividing it into sections. Zone one includes the
thumb, goes up the arm to the central part of the
brain, down the central torso, and down the inner leg
to the big toe. Zone two goes from the second finger, up
the arm to the brain, down the torso (on the outer
edges of zone one), down the leg and into the second
toe. Zones three, four and five follow parallel paths
starting and ending at the third, fourth and fifth
fingers respectively.

The significance of the zones is that whichever parts
of the body exist within a particular zone will be linked
by a flow of energy. This energy can be considered part
of the same energy that permeates all life, indeed all
matter. We are in fact nothing but energy vibrating at
various rates. This energy flows through our bodies as
well as beyond and outside them. Indeed we are aware
of this energy when, for instance, we walk into a room

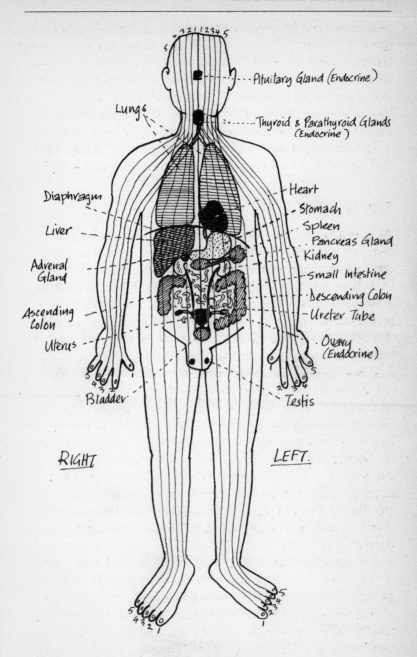

The ten zones of the body, and how they correspond to the main organs and glands.

and sense the atmosphere as one that could be 'cut with a knife'. We sense an energy of tension manifested by those present. Alternatively, if someone is laughing and happy it may 'lift' us to a similar state and help us to forget our problems for a while. This has had a healing effect upon us, and a dynamic of energy has been experienced.

There are various systems of energy flow that can be tapped into. Acupuncture uses a system of meridians, or lines along which the energy is channelled. Reflexology is based on a rather different system whereby the body is divided into zones as described. Where there is a blockage in the flow of this energy (also known as 'ch'i' or 'prana'), then sooner or later some kind of discomfort is experienced. When the blockage is released, energy can flow freely and the body's natural tendency to heal itself and recover its balance can operate. For further discussion of this, see the section of this chapter called 'How does reflexology work?'

The state of one organ within a specific zone may affect the state of another organ in that zone. For example, kidney and eye problems are sometimes linked because the kidney and the eye exist in the same zone (see diagram on page 9).

Transverse zones of the body have also been identified. They were first described by the German reflexologist Hanne Marquardt, who trained with Eunice Ingham. The three transverse zones are shown in the figure opposite, and correspond to the shoulder girdle, the waist and the pelvic floor. Using the longitudinal and transverse zones it is possible to form a sort of grid system on the feet, enabling the reflex points to be very precisely located.

Following on from the principle of the zone system, a connection can also be identified between the right arm and right leg and the left arm and leg – the limbs are seen to have a correspondence with each other. In other words, there is a connection between the right shoulder

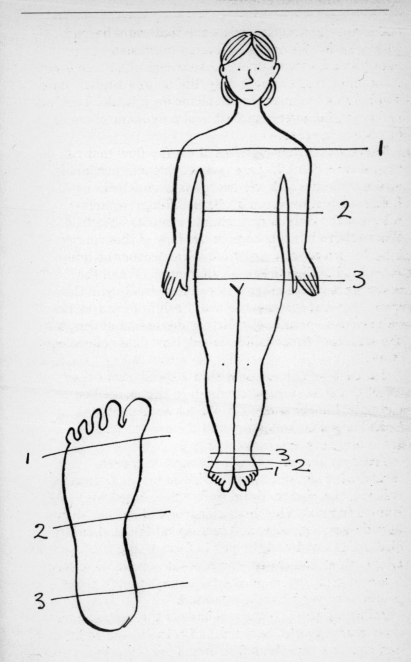

The three transverse zones.

and the right hip, the right elbow and the right knee, the right wrist and the right ankle, the right upper arm and the right upper leg, the right lower arm and the right lower leg, the right hand and the right foot, etc. The same goes for the left side of the body. This is very useful, particularly if it is not convenient or possible to treat a specific part of the body; the corresponding 'cross-reflex' (as it is called) can be treated instead. If, for example, the patient's ankle is badly swollen and sprained, much good work can be done on the wrist to benefit the ankle, when it would have been too painful to treat it directly. Sometimes when a limb has been amputated, so-called 'phantom pains' are experienced in the area where the limb used to be. These pains can be alleviated by treatment using this principle of cross-reflexes. For example, if a foot has been amputated, then treatment of the hand on the same side of the body can be given, and this has been known to relieve the phantom pains experienced in the amputated foot. Similarly, the elbow can be treated by massaging the knee, and also by pressure to the elbow or knee reflex of the foot (and vice versa). The diagram opposite shows the cross-reflexes or 'zone-related areas', as they are also called.

The hands contain all the same reflexes as the feet, but these are not as easily identified, mainly because the hands are smaller and the precise points are harder to find accurately. In my experience, because the feet are usually restricted in shoes, and tend to be neglected, treatment of them is more immediately effective than treatment of the hands, and the sense of well-being induced is more dramatic. Also, our hands are highly cultivated, whereas our feet are in a way more natural, open and 'earthed' – and therefore may be able to tell us about our bodies and our needs with greater clarity.

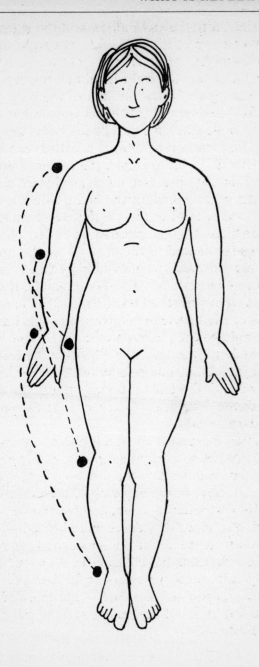

The cross-reflexes or 'zone-related' areas.

WHAT PUTS THE 'REFLEX' INTO REFLEXOLOGY?

A reflex is an involuntary or unconscious response to a stimulus, and this is certainly an appropriate and accurate description of the results of reflexology. We have already described how pressure to particular points in the feet has an effect on parts of the body lying within the same zone. A fascinating and as yet not totally answered question is *how* this mechanism works.

It might be useful at this point to explain a little about reflexes, and how they are used in reflexology. A 'reflex action' occurs in a muscle, gland or organ when an energy current reaches it from the point of stimulus. It is nerve cells or neurons which actually conduct the energy from stimulus to end point, and the reflex response can only occur when that neural pathway is clear.

To understand the reflex nervous system, consider a pinprick to a finger, for example, which will cause the arm to retract from this source of stimulus, without thought. The process happens quite automatically, and is a fast and direct measure to save any further damage or discomfort being caused to the tissue. This is a reflex action.

The autonomic reflex system is responsible for maintaining the internal environment of the body, which includes breathing and heart rate, and governs responses such as sweaty palms that may accompany fear. The brain plays no conscious role in the working of such reflexes – obviously you do not have to be thinking of your breathing for your lungs to operate – though you can breathe more deeply if, consciously, you decide to.

Thus a reflexologist can, through knowledge of the body map on the feet, create a relaxing and healing manipulation along the pathways where autonomic reflexes lie. It is possible in this way for the reflexologist to stimulate internal organs, muscles and glands that would otherwise be beyond reach other than to a surgeon.

As it is electrical impulses that travel along nerves, it is easy to imagine them as channels of energy interconnecting the feet with the rest of the body in the pattern of 'zones' previously described. The reflexologist can detect with their fingers where there are blockages in this energy flow (as explained later in this chapter) by identifying gritty deposits, tender spots, and so on. Specific massage to these points releases blockages and re-establishes a healthy flow of energy, which in turn leads to a healing of the areas which had been dysfunctional.

When certain points on the feet are pressed, the electro-chemical nerve impulse set in motion passes through 'afferent neurons' (neurons carrying messages into the centre) to a ganglion (a clump of nerve cells or neurons standing outside the spinal cord or the brain). From the ganglion the message is taken by 'efferent' neurons (those carrying messages out from the centre) to the specific organ, which will then respond. As mentioned, the nerve impulses initiated by pressing points on the feet seem to be part of the autonomic nervous system, which is primarily concerned with the involuntary action of internal organs, muscles and glands. It seems logical that it is this autonomic system through which reflexology works, because within this system the impulses do not cross over from one side of the body to the other (as would have been the case had they travelled via the brain or central nervous system), and, as we have seen, reflex points on one side of the body refer to parts of the body on that same side.

HOW DOES REFLEXOLOGY WORK?

As already mentioned, we do not know precisely *how* stimulation of particular points on the feet affects specific parts of the body, but that it does affect them has been proved in practice.

The body can be thought of as a universe in its own

right – a system of order and harmony which, when faced with problems or disturbance, will always try to re-establish its balance. There is constant communication within the body, through circulation of the blood, circulation of energy currents throughout the nervous system, and circulation of the vital energy already discussed. The idea of this vital energy is central to reflexology as well as to other ancient healing systems, and it has been called 'life force', 'ch'i' and 'prana', the 'breath of life', that which makes us alive and not dead. It permeates all living cells and all tissue, and follows set paths.

Although the energy paths do not in general correspond to the meridians contacted through acupuncture or shiatsu, the energy is the same. It is as if reflexology uses one key to open a door and other therapies use different keys and different doors. The different doors all lead, however, to the same place in the end, that is, a state of health, balance and well-being.

Although it has not been possible yet to work out scientifically exactly what sort of energy we are talking about here, its existence is indisputable and of fundamental significance to our state of well-being, as many receiving treatment will acknowledge. Kirlian photography, a special form of photographic process through which an impression of the aura, or energy field, surrounding the body is captured on light-sensitive paper, has demonstrated changes in the energy field surrounding the hands and feet after a reflexology treatment. When there is an imbalance in a particular body area the energy field or 'corona' around the relevant reflex area will be diminished. It will become more defined after a reflexology treatment, which shows that the energy has been balanced. This implies, among other things, that some areas will be stimulated to greater activity and others calmed down. Kirlian photography is a useful tool in making visible changes in the energy field surrounding the feet before

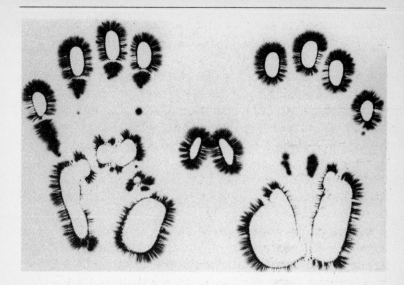

Kirlian photograph of hands.

and after treatment, though it has nothing to do with reflexology or its normal application as such. It is a very immediate way of illustrating the dramatic changes that can result from a treatment – although these will in any case be *felt* by the patient and will manifest themselves in the patient's improved state of health.

As we have seen, the precise workings of reflexology remain something of an enigma. Attempts at scientific explanations have been made, but never seem quite satisfactory. The explanation offered in terms of the autonomic nervous system makes sense to a degree, but no such rational explanations fully encompass the extent of reflexology's effect on the recipient. More than anything, it is the way in which reflexology affects the body's energy (which is itself mysterious) which is its power, and yet it seems almost impossible not only to provide an adequate explanation but even a description of this. However, such an attempt has been made in the following chapters, which provide further insights into this amazing form of healing.

2
A VISIT TO A REFLEXOLOGIST

WHY GO TO A REFLEXOLOGIST?

Perhaps the first question to ask is 'Why go to an alternative practitioner?' People are realizing more and more that conventional Western medicine, which is very much drug-based, does not always provide them with the cures they seek. As alternative therapies gain respectability in our society, people are becoming increasingly aware that they have a choice in the way in which they can be treated. Alternative therapies, being geared towards seeing the person as a whole, inevitably take more time with the patient, and tend to make them feel more personally attended to.

Reflexology has specific qualities which make it very attractive to many people. It is a very simple technique – precise and powerful in its application, but uncomplicated too. All it involves are a pair of hands (the practitioner's) and a pair of feet (yours!). It is highly enjoyable to have the feet massaged and manipulated. It is a relaxing, pampering and enlivening experience all in one, and, as will be shown, can produce extraordinary results.

WHAT CAN I EXPECT AT MY FIRST TREATMENT?

At your first treatment the reflexologist will normally chat to you about your medical history and about any conditions you know you are suffering from or have suffered from in the past. They will probably also ask about various aspects of your life, including your work, family and relationships. In other words, they will be interested in you as a whole person. Although some of this talking may take place before the treatment starts, most of it will come up naturally as your feet are being massaged, because in fact it is the massaging of the feet that tells the reflexologist most about you and that sparks off questions which are most relevant to your situation.

You will be asked to lie down, or perhaps to sit in a special reclining chair with your feet up. You will be asked to remove your shoes and socks (it is appreciated if you have clean feet!), and the treatment will begin.

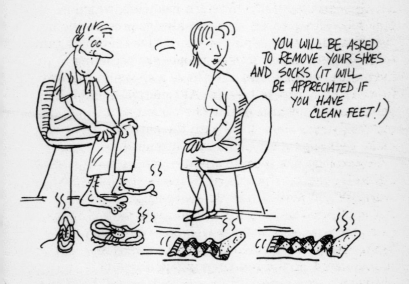

YOU WILL BE ASKED TO REMOVE YOUR SHOES AND SOCKS (IT WILL BE APPRECIATED IF YOU HAVE CLEAN FEET!)

The first treatment will probably last about an hour. The experience of seeing a reflexologist is very different from seeing your GP. Perhaps the most striking difference is the time you will spend together. You will not feel hurried at all, and spending an hour or so focusing on your life and your well-being may be a novel and enjoyable experience for you. The other main difference is that any and all areas of your life may be covered – they are all relevant to the pains and discomforts you may be feeling. A holistic approach is taken, in that you are considered to be much more than your symptoms. Most people feel very nurtured after visiting a reflexologist, not only because of the delightful feeling in their feet, but also because of the interest taken in them.

The practitioner starts with an examination of the feet, noting their temperature, colour, texture, any corns, callouses, blisters, athlete's foot, scars and swelling. If the foot is badly infected with common ailments such as athlete's foot or verrucae, then the corresponding area of the hand can be treated very effectively instead. Likewise, areas with varicose veins are avoided, as pressure on them would probably increase damage and be very painful, but scar tissue can benefit from massage.

Hard skin, corns, and so on may be the result of ill-fitting shoes, or of uneven distribution of the body's weight due to faulty posture. It may be recommended that a chiropodist removes the hard skin, as this makes it difficult for the reflexologist to reach the reflex points. It should be mentioned that chiropody has nothing directly to do with reflexology, but that it can sometimes usefully be used in conjunction with reflexology treatments – as in the case of reflexes which are seriously masked by very hard skin. Often, though, hard skin disappears naturally after consistent reflexology treatments. Whether chiropody is recommended or not really depends on how urgent the reflexologist feels it is to reach deep into the reflex. If you do go to a chiropodist, make sure they are properly qualified and state registered.

As with many aspects of life, there are complex patterns of connection, and of cause and effect, in the feet. On a physical level, if your shoe is uncomfortable, and starts to rub your foot, you will develop areas of hard skin to protect the foot from further damage. What may also happen, however, is that the hard skin over a particular reflex in turn has an effect on the body part connected to the reflex. For instance, a hard patch, caused by bad shoes, over the hip reflex may actually start to create problems in the hip itself. This kind of discomfort or inconvenience would be a signal that the hard skin should be removed. It is therefore worth mentioning that it may be more important than you might have realized to have shoes that fit well, and also to walk barefoot around the house when possible, so that the foot's movement is really unrestricted.

If hard skin develops, it may be there as a protection, and this on more than one level. When a part of the foot is under pressure, and a cushion of hard skin develops, this can be explained at a physical/structural level, that is, as a natural protective mechanism to save underlying tissue from damage (similar to the protective impulse behind blisters). Since different parts of the feet represent different organs and areas of the body, hard protective skin has specific significance according to where it occurs. And because reflexology also works on a symbolic level, emotional connections with the physical conditions can be identified. For example, a hard patch over the inner ear reflex may indicate that you are protecting that area in the sense that you may be avoiding listening to your inner needs. If the reflexologist brings this up in conversation, very often it will spark off a process of unravelling problems which might have been long buried.

If you decide to have areas of hard skin removed by a chiropodist, it may have several possible effects. It will certainly make it easier for the reflexologist to reach the reflexes, and therefore to treat the tender or gritty parts. It will also expose, to varying degrees, the condition which was being protected, and will often bring certain emotions to your conscious awareness, now that the barrier of protection has been removed. If this happens, it means that you are being given the opportunity to contact feelings or traumas which may have been long hidden. Reflexology will help unblock the energy and allow your system to right itself physically and emotionally, giving support to you while you perhaps start to connect with possible *causes* for the problem. If you are not really ready to look at the cause, then your defence mechanism, or protection, will return – in this case, the hard skin will grow again. Usually the change will be gradual, or rather a case of 'two steps forward, one step back'.

Reflexology can treat specific symptoms and can alleviate them. However, because the treatment is a holistic one, not only of the whole body, but also of the whole person, and on many different levels, I find that it works very much by bringing the *cause* of the complaint to the patient's and therapist's conscious awareness. Once this happens, something really permanent can be done to get rid of the complaint. And since no illness is without an underlying cause, any approach which allows the cause to be revealed and understood is to be welcomed, although the extent to which this can happen tends to depend on the intuitive nature of therapist and client.

WHAT DOES THE TREATMENT CONSIST OF?

Before the massage begins some talcum powder is usually applied to the feet, as this makes it easier to move from one point to the next, particularly as the feet often perspire as the treatment proceeds. This is usually considered a good sign, an indication that a healing process has started. If this happens, therefore, there is no need to be embarrassed – the reflexologist will be used to it, and probably pleased!

At first a general massage of the feet is normal, with some gentle manipulation (for instance, rotation of the ankles, and of each toe) to relax the patient. Often the solar plexus reflexes are stimulated at the start of the treatment, again because this has a profoundly relaxing effect and enhances the response to the work on the other reflexes (see diagram on p. 48).

If you have never had a foot treatment before, you may well be feeling a little nervous, as with any new experience, and so the practitioner will be concerned to relax you. Very soon you will start to feel how wonderful it is to have your feet manipulated – we very much neglect them as a rule, and yet, since the whole body is represented on the feet, their neglect is tantamount to neglecting the whole body, be it physical, emotional, mental or spiritual.

The practitioner will then start to work through all the reflex points systematically, alternating deep work with softer, relaxing strokes. The technique used in working on the reflexes is unlike other forms of massage. Usually the thumb is used to apply pressure, but the fingers may also be employed. The thumb is bent at an angle, and the tip is pressed firmly into each reflex point. The reflex points are worked upon with a 'creeping' movement of the thumb, and the next point to be treated is reached. While the thumb is pressing on the reflexes, the other fingers will be gently supporting the foot. The sensations you will experience will vary from one session to the next, according to which areas are out of balance and causing you problems. There is a full discussion of what you will feel in the next section of this chapter.

Each practitioner's treatment will follow a slightly different sequence, and of course variations will occur according to each patient's particular requirements. Usually, however, massage of one foot will begin with the reflexes in the big toe, and then the whole foot will be systematically treated from the toes, across the reflexes on the sole of the foot, down to the heel, and finishing with the reflexes on the sides and top of the foot. The same procedure is then followed on the other foot, although sometimes the practitioner will change from one foot to the other and back again – there are no set rules. Normally, heavy work on the reflexes is interspersed with wringing, stroking and kneading, to aid relaxation. The treatment can include a relaxing breathing exercise, with the reflexologist's thumbs pressing on the solar plexus reflexes of each foot – the patient breathes in as the reflex is pressed, and out as the foot is stretched downwards. This can produce a state of deep relaxation.

Calm, deep breathing from the solar plexus area or stomach area is of course a very useful tool in relaxation. Although breathing exercises are not an intrinsic part of a reflexology treatment, there are times when it can be useful for the reflexologist to help the patient focus on their breathing. An example of this might be at the beginning of a session, to help the patient relax, or indeed at any time if pain or discomfort is experienced during the treatment. 'Going with it' and allowing the breath to continue, not to be held in as is often the tendency, will help to release the discomfort.

There is some argument about which foot to start treatment on. Traditionally, the right side of the body is said to be the active, outgoing, male and externalized side, whereas the left side is receptive, feeling, female and more hidden. According to ancient Chinese philosophy and medicine, two opposite and complementary forces, *yin* and *yang*, make up the totality of existence. The interplay between these two sides of the coin is what is thought to create *ch'i*, or the energy which we have spoken of. It is the balance of *yin* and *yang*, or female and male/left and right sides, which creates good health. Neither side is more important than the other; they are both necessary parts of each of us, male or female. It is often thought preferable to start treatment on a more superficial level first, and get into the deeper levels once the 'ice has been broken' (that is, to start with the right side). A counter-argument, though, maintains that the only way into a person's condition is through the receptive side, and that starting the treatment on the right side might cause the body to reject the stimuli from the massage. Some practitioners alternate one foot with the other, as I have said. By and large, the practitioner feels intuitively what the patient's needs are and how easily receptive or otherwise they may be. My personal belief is that the reflexologist should not stick too rigidly to preconceived ideas about the order of treatment. I have found that starting on the left side usually produces better results, but obviously this is not always the case.

WHAT DOES THE TREATMENT FEEL LIKE?

A word of reassurance should be given to people who feel embarrassed about the state of their feet. Of course it is preferable for you and the reflexologist if your feet are clean at the time of treatment. But apart from this, if there is anything which you might feel awkward about – skin conditions on the feet, deformities or whatever – remember the reflexologist is used to seeing feet of all kinds. That is their job, and anything 'wrong' with your feet is only an indication of an

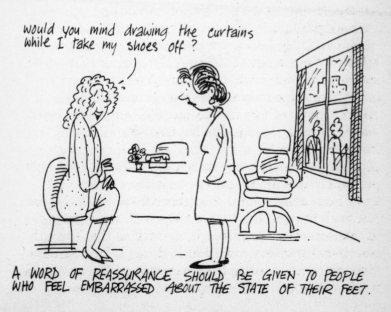

A WORD OF REASSURANCE SHOULD BE GIVEN TO PEOPLE WHO FEEL EMBARRASSED ABOUT THE STATE OF THEIR FEET.

underlying problem which it is the reflexologist's task to uncover. So relax, don't be shy about your feet, and just enjoy the fact that you are now giving them the attention they deserve!

Another common worry among first-time patients is that the treatment will tickle. In fact, the pressure is firm enough for this not to happen – I have treated many people who have sworn that they were unbearably ticklish, and then found that they were not at all. Often ticklishness is an indication of tension, and even if the patient starts the treatment feeling sensitive, soon, when they have relaxed, the ticklish sensation will wear off. Ticklishness may also be an indication to the reflexologist that there is a problem in the area of the body corresponding to the reflex which is ticklish.

It is also natural to feel a bit anxious about whether the treatment will hurt. Certain points may be painful if there is particular imbalance there, but the pain will never last for long, and it can be a 'good' pain in the sense that at a deep level you know that in letting the pain out the underlying problem is being released.

The manipulatory and kneading movements employed by the reflexologist usually feel extremely pleasant and relaxing. The deep thumb pressure applied when working on specific reflexes, however, can give the impression that something sharp is being rubbed into the foot, something not unlike broken glass. Often the patient is sure that the reflexologist is pressing their fingernails into the feet, but this should never be the case, as their nails are kept very short. The sensation of sharpness is in fact the breaking up of certain grainy or crystalline deposits which have accumulated at the reflex points. These grainy deposits can be felt quite distinctly by the reflexologist, and also by the client, as described. No one, however, is quite sure what they are, and it has not actually been possible yet to *see* them (for example at a post mortem). One idea is that the deposits are of some calcium compound, which accumulates at reflexes due to a blockage in energy flow associated with that reflex. It has been suggested that these calcium salts are more easily deposited where there is tension, because tension causes a lessening in the efficiency of all functions in the body, including the ability of the blood to carry its optimum amount of calcium. It is perhaps because of the density of these waste products that they tend to accumulate in the feet.

Another idea is that the deposits accumulate not as a result of blocks in the energy flow, but that the energy flow is blocked because of the existence of the deposits – a chicken and egg situation. We may continue to speculate, and at present it is nothing but speculation, but what is certain is that these deposits exist, because they can be felt, by patient and therapist, and that they can literally be broken up. Through massage, the tiny deposits are crumbled up rather like a sugar lump – you will know this is happening because after a period of massage the gritty sensation, which is a bit like pins and needles, will be gone. Once they are broken up, they can be more easily eliminated, by decomposition and removal via the circulatory systems, urine and sweat glands.

Those areas of the feet which may feel tender are indications to the reflexologist of where the body is most out of balance, and where there may be problems. Occasionally the feet are less sensitive in earlier treatments than later on, as someone who has been fairly unaware of their feet gradually loosens up and becomes more attuned, consciously, to what is going on in their body, and as the major energy blocks are released. Also, with continued treatment, the person's general awareness of themselves, at many levels, will increase, so that fine differences will be felt more easily than before. The whole system is really being purified and refined.

HOW LONG DOES THE TREATMENT LAST?

A treatment session can last anything from half an hour to an hour. Usually, to cover all the reflexes of an adult's feet takes about forty-five minutes, although this obviously varies – if the feet are particularly sensitive, work may have to proceed more slowly. An hour is the usual time allowed, so that neither party feels in any way rushed.

HOW MUCH DOES THE TREATMENT COST?

There is at present no standard cost, but a treatment will usually be between £15 and £20.

HOW MANY TREATMENTS WILL I NEED?

This of course depends entirely on the individual case, but in general, weekly sessions are recommended for the first few weeks at least, after which the client may not feel the need to go so frequently. Often the client *wants* to go for a treatment every week as the effects are so beneficial. It is not normally recommended to have sessions more often than once a week, as the system needs time to readjust and allow the healing process, initiated by the treatment, to evolve before further treatment is applied. There are, however, certain reflexes which can be treated as often as you wish, perhaps by yourself at home – see Chapter 4.

WILL THERE BE ANY AFTER-EFFECTS?

Most people find that they feel very relaxed, and also revived, after a treatment. It is quite common for the patient to fall asleep during a treatment, particularly if it comes at the end of a long day. If you have become this relaxed it is a good idea to try and take things easy for a couple of hours if possible. Some people, however, feel very energized and lively after a treatment, so the best thing is to try and go with whatever your body is telling you, if you possibly can.

There are no dangerous side-effects from reflexology, but in trying to re-establish a healthy balance, and as the energies readjust, various processes may be experienced, which may for a while give the impression that things are a little worse than they had been. This is commonly known as a 'healing crisis'. In the early days of treatment especially, such a healing crisis is often the result of waste matter being expelled, a cleansing or detoxifying process which may feel slightly disconcerting at first. On a physical level, toxins pass into our bodies all the time, via foods with additives, polluted air, and so on, and the body can process and eliminate only a certain amount of these. If levels are very high and/or continue to be absorbed over a long period, then inevitably there will be a backlog of toxins to be eliminated, and the liver, kidneys, bloodstream and lymphatic system will suffer. With a treatment such as reflexology, the body is in a sense given a boost of energy to help the elimination process to work more efficiently.

Therefore, if you do feel that things seem to be getting worse instead of better, a good practitioner should be able to explain that it sometimes takes time for the system to get rid of the 'rubbish' it has been accumulating, normally over years, and to get itself into a finely tuned balance, which is where it naturally wants to go. It is often a case of taking a deep breath and trusting that the process is not always immediate (although, as will be shown, there are many cases in most reflexologists' work where symptoms have indeed disappeared after a single treatment, and have never returned). In fact, if the body is thrown into a degree of turmoil this can be a very good sign – it means the energies have been stimulated to flow more freely, and part of that flowing must necessitate a clearing of any blockages. These blockages manifest themselves as symptoms, what we call 'feeling ill', and when the innate healing forces of the body are encouraged to move and flow, the awareness of these blockages is sometimes brought to the surface. This is experienced as a temporary worsening of the symptom resulting from the blockage, but it is a good sign because it shows that things are moving, without which no cure can be effected.

Most patterns of ill-health have been built up over a very long period, so it is natural that the healing process will also be a gradual one, as layers of problems are allowed to surface and be resolved. However, having said that, it is sometimes remarkable how quickly improvements can be seen (see the case studies on pages 38–40). Sudden changes may also occur in the system, particularly in the resolving of acute conditions such as headaches, toothache, sinus problems and indigestion. According to the tradition of many alternative therapies, recent conditions are considered to be 'nearer the surface', on a mental and physical level, and more quickly healed. Often these are also the acute conditions. Older chronic and persistent conditions are thought to be more deeply embedded (in the psyche also), and to require more time to be resolved. Examples of such conditions include chronic skin conditions such as psoriasis or eczema and long-term digestive difficulties.

How does the body heal itself? The body's natural tendency is towards perfect balance, perfect functioning. When something happens in our lives, be it an emotional or physical disturbance or just perhaps a change in lifestyle, our bodies respond by trying to compensate for the change, and to retain or regain a state of balance. This can be thought of as the body's innate healing mechanism, and the degree to which it will be called into action depends on the degree of disturbance or ill-health. Similarly, when our bodies 'go wrong' this can be seen as an indication that we need to make changes in our lives, for it is the body's way of going about healing us, by grabbing our attention. The more we ignore such signals, the more seriously will we get ill.

Sometimes the body will resist the changes needed to break a pattern, even of ill-health, which it is used to. Change can be frightening. But in the end it is inevitable. Reflexology can be very powerful in encouraging the body to make the necessary changes towards a better state of balance and health.

When our bodies are ill, this can be seen as the final stage, the physical manifestation of a deeper problem which is usually emotional or psychological in nature. If you treat the symptom, and manage to remove it, of course you will feel relief, but if the cause has not been healed then the same symptom or other symptoms will very likely emerge again. In other words, permanent cure can only happen when the cause is dealt with. It may be that all that is necessary is a recognition of, for instance, the unexpressed emotional trauma that caused the stiff shoulder; that in itself may be enough to enable you to let go of the physical signal that something had upset you. Or it may be necessary to do quite a bit of unravelling and work in order to get to the real root of the problem, and so release it.

Here are some examples of ways in which things may *appear* to be getting worse but are actually improving.

Often a healing crisis affects the excretory systems, which may become more active (your body is 'letting go' in more ways than one). Increased activity of the kidneys and bowels are common effects of treatment, and urine and stools may for a time become more smelly. This is a very positive sign, as it indicates that the body is clearing out old toxins.

A seemingly worse cough, looser rather than just a tickle in the throat, or a runny nose rather than a blocked one, may be more of a nuisance for a while and seem more serious, whereas in fact the release of toxins which they indicate is a necessary part of the healing mechanism.

Vaginal discharge may increase for a time, and although this can be unpleasant, it is also often a way of clearing wastes, and shows a shift in energy, which is ultimately part of the healing process.

Skin conditions may erupt more strongly after a foot treatment, but this will be followed by lasting improvement.

Sometimes, diseases which were not properly cured, or rather whose cause was not really worked through, can reassert themselves briefly, again as part of a long-term healing process. An example might be a childhood condition of asthma, which had later in life transmuted to another illness, but which reappears briefly as part of the unravelling process of recovery.

Remember, the reactions described do not necessarily occur at all, but if they do they should be seen as positive indications that the body's healing mechanism is being encouraged to function better, and that a balancing process is occurring within the body. So don't be afraid of these reactions, but do discuss them with your reflexologist, for reassurance and an explanation.

IS REFLEXOLOGY SAFE IN PREGNANCY?

Massage of the feet and reflexology can be very beneficial if you are pregnant. On a physical level, any aches and pains can be greatly relieved, as can conditions such as heartburn and nausea, and on a deeper level, the massage will help you, and of course the baby, to feel nurtured and supported. In fact regular treatments during pregnancy can very much improve the quality of both the pregnancy and the birth. The reflexologist will take great care to give only gentle stimulation of certain points, particularly around the reproductive areas.

IS REFLEXOLOGY OK FOR BABIES AND CHILDREN?

Reflexology can be of great benefit to children, often achieving very quick results, as the child has had less time to accumulate health complications, or at least those layers of ill-health are nearer the surface and therefore more easily peeled away. Children are often more immediately responsive to treatment, because they are less rigid in their ideas and ways, and therefore more open to the healing process.

For a very young baby gentle stroking of the foot will probably be all that is needed, as the feet are extremely sensitive. For older children too the pressure must not be as great as for adult feet. The treatment sessions will also be shorter, partly because it takes less time to cover the reflexes of small feet, and partly because most children will find an hour too long to stay still. Having said that, I have known several children be quite happy to undergo an hour-long session, and even fall asleep, so relaxing did they find it.

SHOULD I TALK TO THE REFLEXOLOGIST DURING A SESSION?

This is entirely up to you. Some people find it very beneficial to have someone to tell their worries to, someone whose undivided attention they have for an hour at a time. If you feel like talking, talk – it can only be of benefit to the healing process. And, of course, anything that you say will be completely confidential.

Sometimes, however, you will be feeling so relaxed that you just want to abandon yourself to receiving the treatment, and you may easily drift off into sleep. If this happens it is probably what you need.

If a particular point is at all painful or having a noticeable effect of some sort on you, it is a good idea to tell the practitioner what you are experiencing, as this may help them and you to get further insight into what is happening.

DO I HAVE TO PREPARE MYSELF FOR THE TREATMENT IN ANY WAY?

No, there is nothing specific you have to do except wash your feet before you come! You might find that as the treatments begin to take effect, your body's natural tendency to want to heal and purify itself will, for example, cause you to alter eating habits, or cut down on smoking. You may not feel the need for so many cups of coffee, and may prefer to drink lots of water instead. (This was my own experience early on in my reflexology treatments.)

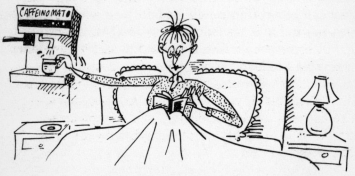

YOU MAY NOT FEEL THE NEED FOR SO MUCH COFFEE ..

The reflexologist may well have suggestions to give you about your diet and lifestyle in general. These will vary from person to person. You may be encouraged to eat more fresh fruit and vegetables, less dairy produce and meat, and perhaps more raw food, but of course each person's needs will be different. Changes in lifestyle could mean anything from going to bed earlier, taking more exercise, moving house, changing job, or reassessing relationships. Your own body will be signalling its needs to you, and the reflexologist can help you to pick up these signals, and perhaps give you one or two pointers as to the best way of responding to your needs. You should find, however, that the treatments themselves will benefit you considerably, even if you make no other conscious changes to the way you live.

CAN OTHER THERAPIES COMPLEMENT REFLEXOLOGY?

Reflexology can combine very well with other therapies, though it is not necessary for it to do so, as it is a very powerful healing tool in its own right. Being in itself a form of massage, it combines perfectly with body massage of various sorts. Shiatsu also works well with reflexology, as does acupuncture. All of these treatments help you to shift energy and heal yourself, so they can be used in combination if you wish. It may be best not to have *too* much going on at the same time, but some people find it helpful to tackle problems from several angles at once. It is really a matter of personal choice, and also of how easily affected you are by the treatment. If you are particularly sensitive to reflexology and are experiencing good and positive results, that is probably quite enough for your system to cope with.

3
CONDITIONS THAT RESPOND WELL

The advantages of reflexology, as of other alternative therapies, lie mainly in the fact that the *whole* system, the whole person – physical, mental, emotional and spiritual – benefits from treatment. There is no doubt that great profit is derived from regular personal attention, physical contact and emotional support. The body's healing mechanism is given a chance to right itself and flow unimpeded. The patient begins to feel, maybe from the very first session (as in my own case after my first treatment), truly in touch not only with their physical body but also, just as importantly, with their emotional and spiritual beings, irrespective of (religious) belief. As a result of the innate healing energy which we can all, without exception, tap within ourselves, many symptoms decline or disappear altogether, sometimes remarkably quickly.

The benefits of reflexology can be manifold, since all parts of the body can be contacted through the reflexes in the feet. Therefore *any* part of the body can in theory (and very often in practice) be helped. Also, as has been suggested, treatment of one organ often benefits another organ lying within the same zone, and treatment of a particular disorder frequently gives relief to another disorder which is in the same zone as the first.

Sometimes reflexology treatment helps in clearing the final stages of a condition which the body has largely healed already. Equally, a treatment can be useful in diagnosing conditions of which the patient is not yet consciously aware. In fact it is a remarkably finely tuned tool for diagnosis, which other alternative practitioners sometimes use for that sole purpose (if you'll pardon the pun!). The practitioner can immediately detect if an area is out of balance, by a temperature difference, dry, flaky or hard skin, feeling the gritty deposits on certain reflexes, or other means.

One other particularly useful aspect of reflexology is its preventative capacity. If used sensitively, it can detect *potential* problem areas, and if these reflexes are worked on many conditions may be prevented altogether. My own observation indicates that it is usually when a specific reflex feels slightly delicate rather than overtly painful that an area of potential rather than actual weakness has been found. To treat preventatively is of course the ideal aim – to encourage the body to be in such fine balance that no manifestation of illness is necessary. Living through the complications of our world, with all its emotional challenges, it is unlikely that we can remain totally free of all symptoms, but a much greater degree of freedom can be achieved if the symptoms are looked on in a sense as friends who are there to tell us that we need to look at the underlying cause, and thereby allow ourselves to grow. As mentioned before, suppressing the symptom will never be a permanent solution; even if that specific symptom does not recur, another will take its place, until the signals of our bodies are really respected and listened to.

The list of conditions that respond well to reflexology is almost unlimited, given our great inner healing potential. However, it is probably true to say that any condition whose cure involves 'clearing' in some way responds most dramatically to reflexology. Here are a few case studies to illustrate the point.

CASE STUDIES

One patient, who had been under some stress and was also overtired, came to me for a reflexology treatment. He was feeling extremely nauseous on this occasion, and his whole abdomen was distended with gas. I worked on the reflexes to the stomach and intestines, as well as giving the feet a relaxing general treatment, and within fifteen minutes his distended stomach had returned to normal and his nausea was gone.

A young lady whose periods had inexplicably stopped came to see me. The reflexes to her uterus and fallopian tubes felt cold and lifeless, and I worked quite deeply on them in the process of giving her general treatments. After several visits, she was feeling much less anxious about her condition, and her energy was greatly boosted. After about two months, her periods began to resume, haltingly at first, and then after a further three months, quite normally. It emerged quite early on that as a child she had suffered from her parents' wish that she had been a boy, and this had manifested itself as a denial of a fundamental part of her femininity much later in life.

A young lady suffering from frequent migraines started on a course of reflexology treatments, visiting the reflexologist at weekly intervals. After an initial increase in the intensity and frequency of the migraines for the first three weeks (a case of a healing crisis), they started easing off, and there were no more attacks after three months of treatments.

A middle-aged lady who had been suffering, at times acutely, from painful sinuses for many years (she had even had them drained twice over the years) came to see me for a treatment. Her sinuses were in fact troubling her on the day, so I did some fairly strong work on them, but the treatment lasted only a short time. After ten minutes or so she commented that the aching pain in her sinuses was lessening, and after twenty minutes that it had completely disappeared. The sinus problem returns very infrequently, and with less strength, and when it does so, a quick treatment relieves the condition. If this lady were to have more regular treatments it is very likely that the sinus problem would disappear altogether.

An elderly gentleman with very bad constipation, from which he had suffered, on and off, all his adult life, was totally cured of the condition after six weeks of reflexology treatments, and is now completely regular for the first time in his life.

A patient suffered from almost constant toothache, although no cavities were identified by his dentist. I did regular work on the reflexes relating to the jaw and neck, and within a month the toothaches stopped. Of course it was not just the specific work on the jaw but also the generally soothing effect of the entire treatment which relaxed him, including his jaw, and so relieved the toothache.

A lady in her early forties came to see me for a treatment. She had undergone major surgery some months before, and was quite weary and lacking in energy, as well as having experienced considerable anxiety. After her first treatment she described feeling as though she were walking on air, and this feeling stayed with her for many days and was renewed each time she had a treatment.

A young woman in her early thirties came to me in a state of great depression and insecurity. She complained that she had a disturbing feeling of not knowing who she really was, a feeling of unreality about her life, her purpose and her personality. She also suffered from frequent headaches, had very dry patches of skin on her arms, legs and back, could not eat properly, and felt, in her own words, 'thoroughly miserable and lost'. She reported to me after her first treatment that she had felt very well, and was greatly encouraged, as results on an emotional and spiritual level were sensed even after a single treatment. She continued to visit me for weekly treatments for six months. Her headaches got worse for a couple of weeks, and then cleared almost entirely (only recurring if she binged on chocolate occasionally!), her skin stopped being rough and dry after about six weeks, and she continued to feel much more balanced and happy. It may also be appreciated how, in this case and many others, the treatment had the effect of allowing the person to open up and talk in a way which they may have found very hard before, and that can be a most powerful release.

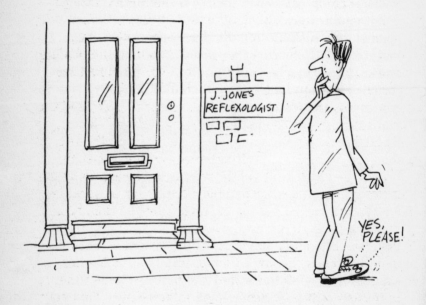

Sometimes people will try reflexology out of a sense of curiosity, even if they have no overt symptoms. The benefits are usually remarkable in terms of the deep relaxation and sense of well-being felt.

Very often people come to have reflexology treatments because they are aware of suffering from a particular disorder, which in fact masks a more important condition within the reflex zone. For example, someone suffering from bad headaches will often benefit from intensive treatment of the digestive system, particularly the colon, and relief of that area will bring about relief of the headaches. In other words the pattern is often more complex, indeed usually so, than we are perhaps conditioned to assume. And, as always, there is an underlying cause for the headaches or digestive problems in the first place. Reflexology is very effective in removing symptoms of all kinds, while at the same time increasing the body's flow of energy and ability to heal itself – which is actually what always happens when a person is healed – and very often puts the person in touch with the cause even without the practitioner saying or asking anything.

Although we can obviously talk about specific conditions which are often successfully relieved by reflexology, there are other levels at which the healing works. For example, traditionally in ancient holistic forms of therapy, the left (*yin*) side of the body represents the female, intuitive, receptive side, and the right (*yang*) side the male, outgoing, active side. Therefore sore points and sensitive areas on the left foot, for example, as well as referring to the specific organs to which they relate, may also be seen to have a significance on a more symbolic level. For example, a sharp pain on the big toe of the left foot at the point relating to the teeth and jaw suggests tension in the jaw, which is often due to its being clenched. People usually clench the jaw in anger and fear, so I would suggest in this instance that the pain in the left toe may represent anger connected with women. This may mean anger at specific women in your life, e.g. your mother, or anger at aspects of yourself as a woman, or at the feminine side of your nature, whether you are a man or a woman. Interestingly, one patient of mine to whom I was about to suggest this very thing started talking about how angry he felt at women a few seconds after I started massaging this point. This is just an example to indicate that there are numerous connections on many different levels, beyond the purely physical, direct association between the reflex points on the feet and the various organs.

This male/female divide, or rather polarity, which I have described applies not only to issues to do with men and women in our lives but also very much to the male and female energies within us. For example, if there is a blockage or problem (anything from a headache to stiff muscles to a broken limb to a tumour) on the right side, it may indicate that the person's active, male side is out of balance. It may be over- or underused, or there may be repression of an emotion – the truth will emerge as the patterns evident in that person's life are explored. In other words, new angles, often highly revealing, can be taken on people's complaints and their possible causes when the situation is viewed also from these intuitive standpoints.

4
'DO-IT-YOURSELF' REFLEXOLOGY

CAN I DO IT MYSELF?

The answer is 'yes, to a certain extent'. A knowledge of the various zones and reflex points of the feet, and an idea of how to work on the reflexes, can at times be very useful, particularly in relieving acute pains such as bad headaches, indigestion, heartburn or stomach cramps, and also of course in generally relaxing the feet. If the foot is given a good massage, remember this is like the whole body receiving a massage.

It should be noted, however, that treating yourself cannot really compare with having a proper treatment from a qualified practitioner. This is because, firstly, the good practitioner knows exactly what they are doing, and can be extremely precise in treating the appropriate areas, and secondly, part of the benefit of being treated by someone else is the very fact that it is someone else. The reflexologist acts, among other things, as a channel. By channelling I mean that the reflexologist is an intermediary, bridging the blockage. If ignored, the blockage may lead to ailments of varying degrees of severity or may be experienced, for example, as lack of motivation or inspiration, and a general lethargy about all aspects of our lives. Although the main work is in stimulating the body's internal energy system and helping it to flow unimpeded, there are times when the practitioner is actually channelling off, or grounding, energy from the patient. Most of us are aware these days of suffering from some sort of stress or tension. Our lives are very pressured, because of, for instance, working to strict timetables, getting stuck in traffic jams, being late for appointments, and so on. The reflexologist may be seen as channelling off 'negative' energy, although the term is slightly misleading. The energy is not exactly negative, but rather there is a blockage in its flow, or a build-up at certain reflexes, which the practitioner is able to sense and to filter off.

This book does not aim to provide an extensive set of instructions on how to do reflexology, but some guidelines about ways in which you can treat yourself, with particular suggestions for ways to relieve certain common conditions.

DO I NEED TO PREPARE MYSELF IN ANY WAY?

There is nothing special that you need to do; if you urgently need to treat a particular reflex, you can do that through your socks or tights fairly successfully. However it is better, if you can, to have bare feet, because you have easier access to the reflexes, and it is good for the foot to feel free and to be able to breathe. You should sit comfortably, so that in reaching for your foot you are not straining your back. Ideally you should bend one knee and put your foot on your lap, so that you can see as much of the sole of the foot as possible. However, if this is too uncomfortable for you, don't worry, it is not essential, and once you become familiar with the position of the reflexes, all you need do is feel them with your fingers. Indeed it is often the case that you develop greater sensitivity in your fingers when you are not looking, as of course is evident with blind people. If it is too difficult to reach certain parts of the feet, don't forget that the corresponding points on the hands can be treated very effectively too. So get yourself into whatever position is most comfortable, and start the massage. Here is a suggested routine for

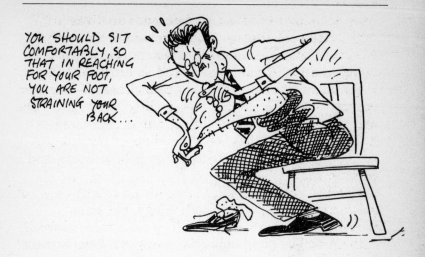

YOU SHOULD SIT COMFORTABLY, SO THAT IN REACHING FOR YOUR FOOT, YOU ARE NOT STRAINING YOUR BACK...

a general self-treatment, and then a list of some of the most common conditions and how to relieve them.

(1) It is a good idea to start by placing the ball of your thumb on the solar plexus reflex (where a great deal of tension is stored) and pressing into the reflex with a gently rotating movement for a minute or two. By relaxing the solar plexus, you are able to breathe more easily and deeply, instead of breathing just from the top of your lungs. By relaxing the solar plexus area it is easier for the bottom of the lungs to expand, which releases tension at a deep level, and makes response to further treatment more effective.

(2) Hold the ankle firmly with one hand and with the other rotate the foot, first in one direction and then in the other. Make sure you are not letting your foot do the work. The foot should be as relaxed and passive as possible, and the hands should do all the work. Continue this for about a minute, or as long as it feels pleasant. If the ankle is very stiff try and continue this loosening exercise until you feel the stiffness lessen. If it is very painful, don't force anything – you will know how much you can take – and this applies to all of the following techniques.

(3) Now hold the base of the big toe and rotate the toe with your fingers. Hold the base of the toe firmly so that there is some resistance against which to do the rotation. Rotate first in one direction and then in the other, as with the ankle. Repeat with each toe.

(4) Take each toe, one at a time, and with your thumb and finger(s) pull gently, and then more firmly. Pull straight out in the direction in which the toes are pointing. Do not pull them out at an angle, unless you are sure that your toes are very flexible and that you won't hurt yourself. If the toes crack, that is fine, but you should not force them to do so.

(5) With one hand hold the top of your foot to steady it, and with the other hand make a fist. Place your fist on the ball of your foot and stroke all the way down the sole of your foot. Return your fist to the ball of your foot and start again. Repeat as many times as feels appropriate – I would suggest at least half a dozen times in any case, as this has a powerfully relaxing effect not only on the foot itself but on the whole body. The effect is like massaging the whole of the torso, and is very beneficial. Some of the reflex points for internal organs such as the liver and kidneys may feel tender (this is very common), so, again, use your judgement about how hard you want to press. A certain degree of sensation, when stimulating the reflexes, is of course to be expected, as the body's energies are frequently out of balance, but if the pain is extreme you should see a reflexologist in any case. (As already said, doing reflexology on yourself, though it can certainly have beneficial results, is in no way a substitute for a proper treatment.)

A word should be said here about one of the most frequently used techniques in reflexology. This involves using a bent thumb, and pressing the tip of the thumb into the part to be treated, and then

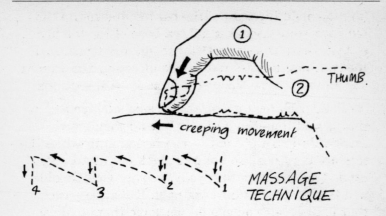

creeping with the thumb rather like a caterpillar along the line of the reflex (see the diagram above). The thumb thus straightens and bends and straightens again as it moves along the part to be treated. This technique takes a bit of practice, but you can do quite a lot of good even if you haven't got it absolutely right. The really deep work will probably be done by a reflexologist anyway. The idea is to go in deep enough to feel the crystalline deposits and help break them up, so there is not a great deal of point in being too gentle, but if the treatment you give yourself is largely for relaxation, that is fine.

(6) Place your thumb and forefinger on either side of the space between the big and second toes, where the toes join the rest of the foot. Now with a pinching action creep up the foot between the two bones as far as you can, and then slide back down, giving a little pinch at the base of the toes. Repeat. Then proceed to do the same movement between the next two toes, and so on, until the whole foot has been covered. This has the effect of clearing out the lungs and aiding lymph drainage.

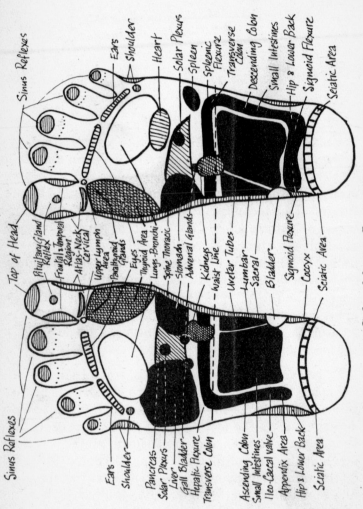

Sole of foot reflex areas.

Sinus Reflexes

Ears
Shoulder
Heart
Solar Plexus
Spleen
Splenic Flexure
Transverse Colon
Descending Colon
Small Intestines
Hip & Lower Back
Sigmoid Flexure
Sciatic Area

Top of Head
Pituitary Gland Reflex
Frontal & Temporal Region
Atlas-Neck Cervical
Upper Lymph Area
Parathyroid Glands
Eyes
Thyroid Area
Lungs-Bronchi
Spine Thoracic
Stomach
Adrenal Glands
Kidneys
Waist Line
Ureter Tubes
Lumbar
Sacral
Bladder
Sigmoid Flexure
Coccyx
Sciatic Area

Sinus Reflexes

Ears
Shoulder
Pancreas
Solar Plexus
Liver
Gall Bladder
Hepatic Flexure
Transverse Colon
Ascending Colon
Small Intestines
Ileo-Caecal valve
Appendix Area
Hip & Lower Back
Sciatic Area

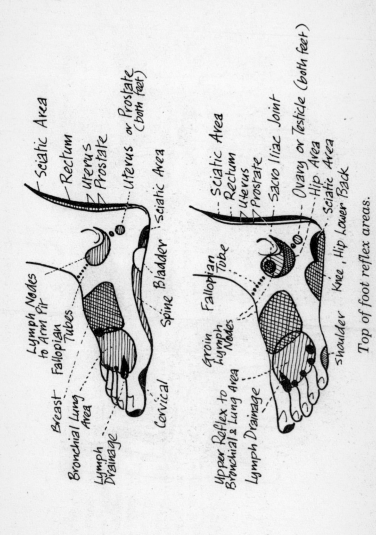

Sciatic Area
Rectum
Uterus or Prostate
Uterus or Prostate (both feet)
Sciatic Area
Lymph Nodes to Arm Pit
Fallopian Tubes
Breast
Bronchial Lung Area
Lymph Drainage
Spine
Bladder
Sciatic Area
Cervical

Sciatic Area
Rectum
Uterus
Prostate
Sacro Iliac Joint
Ovary or Testicle (both feet)
Hip Area
Sciatic Area
Fallopian Tube
Groin Lymph Nodes
Upper Reflex to Bronchial & Lung Area
Lymph Drainage
Shoulder
Knee, Hip Lower Back

Top of foot reflex areas.

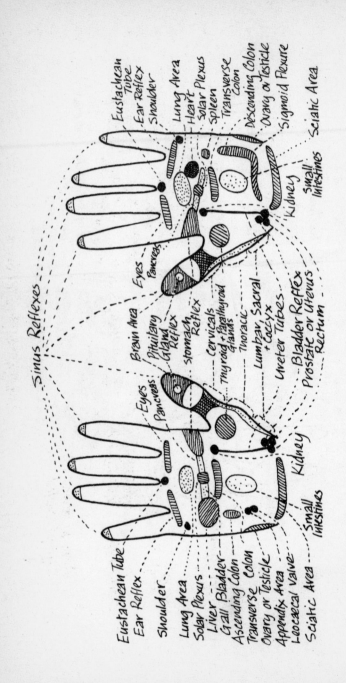

Palm of hand reflex areas.

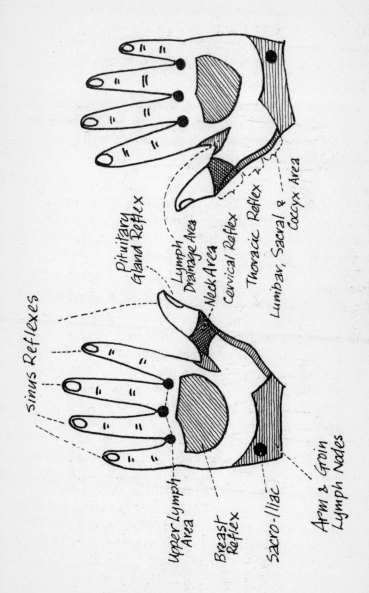

Back of hand reflex areas.

Sinus Reflexes

Pituitary Gland Reflex

Lymph Drainage Area

Neck Area

Cervical Reflex

Thoracic Reflex

Lumbar, Sacral & Coccyx Area

Upper Lymph Area

Breast Reflex

Sacro-Iliac

Arm & Groin Lymph Nodes

SOME SPECIFIC CONDITIONS YOU CAN TREAT YOURSELF

The reflexes mentioned below should be pummelled fairly deeply by your thumb (this is the easiest way), either by pressing the thumb into the reflex and rotating it, or by the creeping movement described.

Abscess
An abscess can be brought to a head by massage of the relevant reflex, and once this has happened, it is on the way to being healed. Subsequent massage will accelerate the healing process.

Acne
Massage should be given to the reflexes of the parts affected, and also to the reproductive areas, digestive areas, liver, solar plexus, kidneys, pituitary, thyroid and adrenals, spleen and lymph ducts.

Addiction
Whether the addiction is to drugs, alcohol or food, the support of a professional reflexologist, among other people, would of course be of greater help than working on your own, but there is a useful amount of back-up work which you can do. This is particularly helpful in encouraging you to nurture and value yourself. A general massage is of great help in relaxing you, so cover whichever reflexes feel they need it. Because of the strain the addiction will have caused to your physical system, particular attention should be given to the reflexes of the liver, kidneys, adrenals, circulatory system and parathyroids (which are of great help in relieving muscle cramps). Relief from the effects of the build-up of toxins in the muscle tissues can be gained by massaging the reflexes to the parts of the body which are causing particular pain.

Allergies
Give massage to the reflexes of any specific body parts affected, and also to the solar plexus, pituitary,

lymphatics, adrenals and spleen. In the case of food
allergies, particular attention should be given to the
digestive areas too.

Anxiety
An overall massage of the feet is of great benefit, but
specific attention can be given to the kidneys, adrenals,
the solar plexus and the heart reflexes. Also, if
discomfort is felt in any particular part of the body, for
example the stomach, during periods of anxiety, then
that reflex too should be worked upon.

Arthritis and rheumatism
Arthritis causes pain and inflammation of the joints;
rheumatism includes pain, stiffness and swelling of
muscles and joints. The conditions have quite a
profound effect on the whole body, apart from just the
specific areas, so a good general treatment is necessary.
However, give special attention to the joints and
muscles affected, and to all zone-related areas (for
instance, elbow for knee), as well as to the pituitary,
parathyroids, kidneys, solar plexus, adrenals,
bronchials and lungs.

Asthma
Concentrated massage should be given to the reflexes
of the lungs and bronchi. Work should also be done on
the solar plexus, spine, adrenals, pituitary, thyroid,
reproductive glands, heart and ileo-caecal valve.

Cancer
The term 'cancer' refers to malignant growths in the
body. It is thought that there is an emotional
component to the origin of such growths, and that they
come about when a feeling or feelings are not
expressed, for example anger or grief. Reflexology can
help both by calming and relaxing you, and also by
allowing you to bring up and express, literally to 'let
out', what you have been blocking. There are many
cases of people curing themselves of what had been

diagnosed as cancer, so it does not need to be a death sentence. Apart from a general relaxing massage of the whole foot, you should concentrate on the specific body parts affected by the cancer, and also work on the lymphatic areas and the spleen. Again, great benefit may be had by visiting a professional reflexologist, as well as trying many other forms of natural healing.

Circulatory problems

A general massage of all reflexes helps the circulation of the blood to the whole body. Chilblains on the feet and hands can frequently be greatly relieved. Varicose veins may be difficult to heal, but treatment (on the feet, not on the veins themselves) should stop things from getting worse. Massage should be given to the reflexes of the areas affected, and also the heart, intestines and liver.

Common cold

Thoroughly massage the reflexes of the nose, throat, lungs, eyes, ears and all parts of the head. The sinus reflexes should also be worked upon. If the cold is especially severe, and you have a fever too, work on the reflex of the pituitary gland as often as you can while the fever persists.

Conjunctivitis

This condition involves inflammation of the membrane lining the eyelids, swelling and discharge from the eye. Massage should be given to the eye reflexes, upper lymph nodes, kidneys, adrenals and upper spine. Because this is an inflamed condition, it is worth trying the point on the heel mentioned under 'Inflammation' (page 60). It should also be noted that, being an 'angry' condition, conjunctivitis can often be caused by a feeling (usually unconscious) of anger, so it is important, as always, to try and look to the cause.

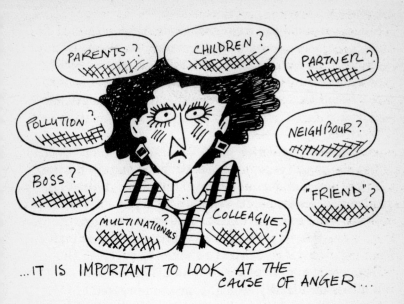

...IT IS IMPORTANT TO LOOK AT THE CAUSE OF ANGER...

Constipation

Start working on the right foot, at the base of the ascending colon. Press up the colon reflex with the thumb, using the creeping movement described, and then continue moving across, following the transverse colon until you reach the inner edge of the foot. Then transfer to the left foot, continuing along the reflex for the transverse colon. Press firmly and slowly all along the reflexes. Stop at the junction point between the transverse and descending colon. Now place your thumb on the anus point; work back along the descending colon to the junction of the transverse colon, and then back down firmly to the anus point. This has the effect of unblocking the large intestine, and should, after a couple of treatments, relieve the constipation.

It is worth noting that constipation is often an indication of 'holding on' in both a literal and symbolic way – perhaps showing a reluctance to let go of old patterns and habits. Conversely, diarrhoea can be seen as 'letting go'.

Cramps

Muscle cramps are frequently caused by lack of calcium in the muscle. Work should therefore be done on the reflexes to the parathyroids, as these distribute calcium through the body. Also massage the reflexes to the areas affected by the spasms, and the heart reflex.

Cystitis

This bladder infection often causes a burning sensation during urination, sometimes with a constant desire to empty the bladder. Massage the bladder, kidney, ureter tubes, adrenals, pelvic lymph nodes, pituitary and prostate reflexes. Lower back pain is often experienced with cystitis, so massage the spine reflexes as well.

Depression

Depression usually stems from a suppressed or repressed emotion, perhaps anger, grief or joy. An overall general treatment will induce a sense of well-being and relaxation, and help these repressed emotions to come out, and of course once they are out, then you will relax even more.

Earache

Massage to the ear reflexes should be given, as well as to the side of the head, neck and upper spine, the Eustachian tubes and upper lymph nodes.

Eczema

This is often an allergic reaction, and is also very much stress-induced. Massage should be given to the reflexes of all affected parts, and to the pituitary, adrenals, kidneys, digestive areas, liver and solar plexus.

Eye disorders

Massage the reflexes to the kidneys, solar plexus and stomach as well as the eye reflexes. The kidneys lie in the same zone as the eyes, and disorders of one are often linked to disorders of the other.

Fatigue

This can result from stress, whether physical, emotional or mental, so a similar approach to the one you would adopt for treating stress would be appropriate (see page 64). It may be worth pointing out here that a holistic understanding of fatigue may reveal that it is often a way of avoiding something that is uncomfortable or painful to look at.

Fractures

Reflexology can help the healing of a broken bone if massage is given to the reflex point of the affected area, as well as the zone-related area (for instance, ankle for wrist, shoulder for hip). Also massage the reflexes to the spine, adrenals, solar plexus and parathyroids. The body's healing mechanism will be stimulated to work towards its maximum in this way.

Gallstones

Treatment can help small gallstones to be passed, by massage of the gall bladder reflex, bile duct (which links the duodenum to the gall bladder), small intestine, liver, solar plexus and adrenals. If gallstones have been removed by surgery, massage to the reflex can greatly reduce the tenderness felt around the scar tissue, and will generally accelerate the healing process.

Gassiness

You should work on the reflexes of the stomach, the ileo-caecal valve (near the base of the ascending colon) and the sigmoid flexure (at the base of the descending colon near the rectum). Massage of the solar plexus, diaphragm and liver may also be useful.

Gout

This painful condition of the joints (usually the fingers and toes) can be helped by massage to the affected area. If the big toe, for example, is gouty, then the thumb could be treated. Also treat the solar plexus, kidneys, liver, adrenals, parathyroids and pituitary.

Haemorrhoids
Massage should be given to the reflex of the anus, the intestines, rectum, lymph circulation, liver, heart, solar plexus and adrenals.

Hay fever
This allergic reaction to pollen can cause a runny nose, sore and itchy throat, watering eyes and sneezing. Reflexology to the sinuses, nose, eyes and throat, as well as the adrenals, head and digestive areas, can greatly help.

Headaches
A good idea is to start with firm rotation of the big toe, which has the effect of loosening the neck. Then proceed to a strong pressure on all the reflex points for the head occurring on the big toe. Some of these will probably feel quite sharp. Try to persist with the massage anyway. The best method to use is the same creeping motion with the thumb described earlier, gradually working your way all over the underside and tip of the big toe.

Another very powerful point for getting rid of headaches is on the hand. With the thumb and index finger of one hand pinch the fleshy part of the other hand between the thumb and index finger (see diagram opposite). Find the part that feels particularly tender and manipulate and massage it as hard as you can bear. This is one of the most effective cures for headaches, and is very easy to apply. Do it on both hands, but if the headache is on one side more than the other, concentrate on that side.

Of course headaches can be caused by many things. On a physical level, for example, they may be due to a malfunction of the liver, or of the digestive system, so there will be occasions when the reflexologist would

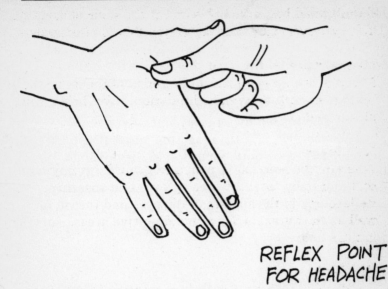

REFLEX POINT
FOR HEADACHE

also concentrate treatment on these other areas.
Therefore, if your headache is not relieved by the
methods suggested above, it might be an idea to give
yourself a general treatment as far as you can, so that
you cover other reflexes which may be connected with
the headaches. Many headaches are caused by
eyestrain, earache or sinus problems, so it is certainly
worth working on these reflexes too.

Heartburn

This is usually caused by contraction of the oesophagus
muscles, when acid from the stomach flows back into
the oesophagus. The reflexes to the oesophagus and
chest area should be massaged, as well as those of the
stomach, solar plexus and adrenal glands.

Hernias

These usually occur in the groin (inguinal hernia) and
where the oesophagus passes through the diaphragm
(hiatus hernia). Massage should be given to the
affected reflex, and also to the solar plexus and
adrenals.

Hiccoughs

These are spasms in the diaphragm, therefore massage should be given to the reflexes of the diaphragm, as well as to those of the solar plexus and the pituitary.

High blood pressure (hypertension)

This may be caused by tension, being overweight, alcohol, smoking, and too much tea and coffee. Symptoms may be quite varied, and may include headaches, nose bleeds, dizziness, insomnia, blurred vision, noises in the ears, and shortness of breath. Massage should be given to the heart reflex, the solar plexus, adrenals, kidneys, eyes, lungs, head, neck and spine.

Incontinence

This involves a problem with the bladder, usually weak bladder muscles. With children, and bedwetting, this is often the result of emotional disturbance. Reflexology can not only help the condition, but can also encourage the cause to surface. Massage the bladder reflexes, the kidneys, ureter tubes, solar plexus, adrenals, spine, prostate and pituitary.

Indigestion

This may also be accompanied by gas in the stomach and intestines. It is a good idea to start by running your fist several times down the sole of the foot, from under the toes down to the heel, which, in effect, relaxes the whole of the torso. Then work on the stomach and intestine reflexes, and on the solar plexus and diaphragm.

Inflammation

It has been found that inflammation of any part of the body can be helped by pressing a point on the soles of the feet where the arch and ball of the heel meet.

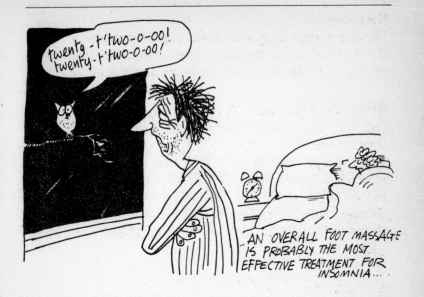

twenty-t'two-o-oo! twenty-t'two-o-oo!

...AN OVERALL FOOT MASSAGE IS PROBABLY THE MOST EFFECTIVE TREATMENT FOR INSOMNIA....

Insomnia

An overall foot massage is probably the most effective treatment, to be done in bed before you want to sleep. As you get more relaxed, gentle stroking, especially over the tops of the feet, induces a very sleepy state. Of course this is another situation where treatment by another person would probably have an even better effect, but you can help yourself quite a bit none the less.

Kidney stones

These are deposits of a calcium salt in the kidneys. The idea is to try and locate the stone on the reflexes and then to move it from the kidney reflex to the bladder via the ureter. Massage should also be given to the pituitary, thyroid and parathyroids. (Massage of the kidney reflexes helps all kinds of kidney disorders and infections, and also water retention.)

Low blood pressure (hypotension)

With this condition, you may feel very tired and extremely sensitive to cold and heat, and your pulse may race after only slight exertion. Sometimes, too, there will be a feeling of greater tiredness in the morning than before going to bed. Massage the heart reflex, solar plexus, kidneys, head, brain and adrenals.

Menopause

Possible problems encountered at this time are hot flushes, dizziness, severe headaches, digestive problems and heavy, irregular periods. Useful points to treat are the ovaries, fallopian tubes, uterus, pituitary, adrenals, thyroid, head, ears and digestive areas. (Massage of the adrenals and pituitary can produce a hormone supplement which softens the discomfort.)

Menstrual problems

These may include heavy, scant, irregular or painful periods, pre-menstrual tension, or an absence of periods altogether. Massage should be done on the ovaries and uterus reflexes. A week before the period is due, it is also good to massage the reflexes of the pelvis, the lymph glands, the lumbar vertebrae and the sacrum (the lower section of the spine where much tension is stored). Connected reflexes which may encourage regular, normal periods are the pituitary, thyroid, adrenals, solar plexus, head and fallopian tubes.

Mucus

Excess mucus can be alleviated by massage to the reflexes of the adrenals and the ileo-caecal valve.

Pregnancy

Particular care should be taken, especially early on in the pregnancy, but great benefit in terms of relaxation can be achieved by massage to the entire pelvic region. This stimulates circulation, and can help to make both the pregnancy and the birth easier. Specific conditions within pregnancy such as morning sickness, constipation and heartburn can be helped by massage to the appropriate reflexes. Be careful to avoid any real pressure to the uterus point; massage should in general be gentle, especially if you are doing it yourself.

Scars
Scar tissue can diminish considerably with regular massage to the reflexes of the affected parts. Recent scars may disappear more easily than old ones, but good results have eventually been attained even with very old scars.

Sciatica
Pain of the inflamed sciatic nerve can be felt anywhere from the lower back to the buttocks, the back of the thigh and either behind or above the knee. Treatment should be given to the sciatic reflex across the heel of the foot and to the area up the back of the ankle and calf, as well as to the lower spine, sacro-iliac joint, pelvis, hip and knee.

Sexual problems
These are often related to emotional problems, and since reflexology is very effective in increasing people's awareness of their underlying emotional state, it can be of considerable help in relieving various problems of sex (even on a mechanical level) and of sexuality in its broader context. Therefore a general massage is recommended, perhaps with particular attention to the reflexes which help anxiety, depression and stress (see under these headings). Of course massage to the reflexes of the sex organs will also help their integration with the whole person. Although there is quite a bit you can do to help yourself here, it should be emphasised that interaction with a trained practitioner will of course give you a feeling of support which you may need, as well as the expertise of their training.

Shingles
Provided the reflexes corresponding to the affected parts are not too tender to touch, reflexology can be of

great help in alleviating this painful condition. It is also particularly helpful in relieving the pains which sometimes linger after the blisters themselves have healed. Massage is given to the reflexes of the affected areas, and also to the lymphatic areas, solar plexus and spleen.

Stiff neck

The big toe should be gently rotated for a few minutes, as this releases the neck, and then firm massage should be given down the side of the big toe next to the second toe. Neck problems can lead to pain in the shoulder, arm and back and to headaches and ear problems. Massage should therefore also be given to the reflexes of the cervical spine, shoulder, arm, head, ears, solar plexus, adrenals and the lymphatic system.

Stress

A general massage of the feet will relax you, but you could pay particular attention to the solar plexus, head and heart reflexes, and to any specifically painful area (for instance the shoulders, where the muscle may be knotted).

Toothache

This can be relieved by massage to the teeth reflexes (which include the gums) and to the face and solar plexus. Of course, if the toothache persists, you should visit a dentist. Stiffness of the jaw can cause aching teeth, so massage of all the face and head reflexes will help, as will the relaxing effect of a general massage.

Ulcers

Most commonly these occur in the stomach (gastric/peptic ulcer) and the small intestine (duodenal ulcer). Massage should therefore be given to the appropriate reflex, and also to the solar plexus, diaphragm, adrenals and heart.

Water retention
Give massage to the adrenal, heart and kidney
reflexes. Also massage the specific reflex points for
those parts of the body which are swollen.

5
THE HOLISTIC APPROACH TO HEALTH

Indications of what a holistic approach to health implies have been given throughout this book, but this chapter will expand on these ideas, and try to develop some of the issues further.

HOW DOES A HOLISTIC APPROACH DIFFER FROM CONVENTIONAL MEDICINE?

In broad terms, alternative therapies are biased towards a holistic approach, which basically means that the patient is seen as a whole human being. Thus, all aspects of their life are taken into account. The holistic practitioner will want to enquire about the patient's lifestyle and habits, personal problems, emotional state, diet, childhood and so on, including some medical history. The practitioner will thus be able to piece together a detailed picture of that person, a rounded human being who happens to have developed certain symptoms. The patient is never clumped together with other people who have the same symptoms in an arbitrary way, as each case is always unique, just as we are all unique. Certain patterns of ill-health may emerge, and there may of course be similarities between individual cases, but each person is essentially a special case.

In conventional Western medicine, patients tend to

be seen as a collection of symptoms to which a name is then given. The main aim, then, is to remove the unpleasant symptoms, and rarely, if ever, are their causes focused upon. Often strongly suppressive drugs are used to mask the symptoms, but what is often not realized is that the location of the symptoms may indicate the area of the body which either physically or symbolically represents the area of your life which needs attention. Therefore conventional medicine and alternative medicine can be seen as being complementary in the overall treatment of the symptoms and cause of illness. Because most of us have been brought up with Western medicine, we have a strong belief in it, and certainly there are times when it is much simpler to treat a condition by conventional means. Often it is only when conditions become life-threatening that people start to consider their root.

Although a therapy like reflexology is often used to relieve painful conditions, it does not do so in a suppressive way. It stimulates the body's innate healing mechanism, re-establishing an undisturbed flow of energy or vital force. It is a gentle but often strikingly effective encouragement towards good health, not a bullying, forceful one, which may ultimately cause the body to rebel further.

RESPONSIBILITY FOR OUR OWN HEALTH

This is probably one of the key issues for anyone undergoing an alternative form of therapy. In the West we have, by and large, been conditioned to believe, or at least hope, that 'the doctor will make it better'. Of course it is natural to want the nasty pain to go, but what we don't realize until it is pointed out is that (a) the pain is nasty because it is trying to tell us something, and (b) we have the innate ability to heal ourselves of any pain or disease. And it is here that the practitioner can help so much to highlight our situation for us.

Although it may at first seem daunting to feel that we can actually take responsibility for ourselves, in the end it is the only lasting answer. Alternative medicine has a real understanding of this, and gives every encouragement to the patient to help themselves in every way, while using the particular tools and skills at its disposal to accelerate the process. The process in this case can ultimately be seen as the development of the natural realization of our innate ability to love ourselves on all levels.

LOVING OURSELVES

In Western society, modesty tends to make us forget this basic principle, and we confuse this love with being egotistical, selfish or arrogant. We enter, at an early age, the vicious circle of misunderstanding which produces disorder and hence illness. However, since these misperceptions have been learnt, they can also be un-learnt.

To expand on this further, it is true I think to say that our society and the way most of us have been parented do not encourage us to learn to be responsible for ourselves. As young babies and children we are quickly taught to be dependent on our parents to tell us what is right and what is wrong, and particularly what feelings are acceptable or not. This is not the result of conscious design, but of disciplinarian parenting which does not allow the child to trust their own feelings. Young children are far nearer the truth of their feelings and their needs than adults realize – and they can only come to accept and love themselves if the messages they get from their parents are that they are deeply and unconditionally loved and accepted by them. Young children *need* to express and develop their ego; if this is not allowed to happen, where the ego is not allowed to flow along the true channels of that child's inner design, then the child will grow up frustrated in their unexpressed ego needs, and will

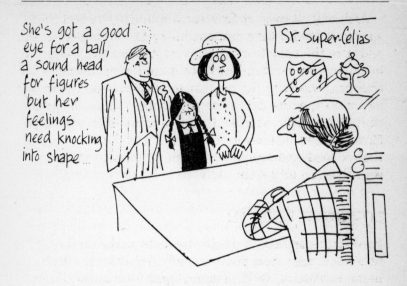

essentially remain a child emotionally. This has of
course happened to virtually all of us to some extent
and it is recognizing the child within, and parenting it
lovingly ourselves, that allows us to bring ourselves
back to wholeness.

Time spent receiving a treatment such as reflexology
is a wonderful doorway to that process, as it unlocks so
many patterns and emotional responses which may
have been long hidden.

TIME WITH THE PRACTITIONER

Unfortunately one of the most frustrating aspects of
most people's visits to their GP is the short time
available for the consultation. GPs are under such
pressure that they just cannot spare more than five or
ten minutes with each person, so the system does not
allow for a more overall approach to the patient, their
life and underlying problems, even when the doctor
would like to be able to investigate some of these
issues. The emphasis is placed rather, as we have said,
on removing the unwelcome symptom.

The difference in symptoms disappearing as a result of one of the alternative therapies is that we are working with the body's own natural healing mechanisms, and the body will heal itself and put itself through whatever healing crises are necessary only as fast as it can handle the process, and only to the extent that it is able to unravel the network and many layers of difficulty (physical, emotional, mental and spiritual) that it has experienced. It is one of life's greatest satisfactions to get through these inhibiting problems and arrive at our true selves.

Modern medicine has become almost a religion, in the sense that if something is 'wrong' in our lives we turn to the 'magic' of drugs or surgery. However, modern drugs often have side-effects, and can create new health and life problems. So in a sense one problem is frequently replaced by another. It is often because of such experiences, though, that people begin to turn to alternative or complementary treatments.

All of us are capable of good health and productive lives, not merely a lucky few. When we are faced with difficulties in our lives, our path is made much easier if we can begin to see these difficulties as messages that there are things we can do to improve our situation. In other words, if we can look at ill-health as a process leading towards potential improvement in the quality of our lives and greater insight into the self, we will see ourselves less as poor victims of an unpleasant disorder, which interrupts what we want in life, and more as the very instruments of our own cure.

What we really need is an adjustment of our beliefs, and a desire to cure the disorder at its root, that is, to heal the cause. This will enable us to return to health with a deeper understanding of what will bring satisfaction into our lives. By expanding our awareness of our body, mind and spirit, we will grow towards a better understanding of our own power to heal ourselves and cope with the stresses of modern life.

A good start is to consider our problems as

challenges, challenges to which there are always solutions, which will help us to realize that there is light at the end of the tunnel. All of us are equipped with the tools to deal with such challenges, and alternative therapies such as reflexology can play their part here.

ALTERNATIVE THERAPIES AS PREVENTATIVE TREATMENT

One of the key aspects of alternative therapies and a holistic approach to health is that very often the treatment turns out to be preventative. This is certainly very much the case with reflexology. It is preventative in two ways. Firstly, it is possible, by the minute investigation of the foot reflexes, for the practitioner to find areas which may be potential problem areas, even if they are not already so. This may be indicated by a feeling of tenderness in the reflex, striking temperature differences between different areas of the feet, and many other signs. Secondly, it is preventative because, once areas of potential weakness have been identified, work can be done on them so as to stimulate the body's healing forces to flow unimpeded, and thus to avert the particular condition which was likely to develop.

MORE THOUGHTS ON ALTERNATIVE MEDICINE

The term 'alternative' has come to be used for any fringe medicine that veers away from the mainstream of work done by medics in the West, and it is often practised by people with no formal medical training. In reality, it is Western medicine which is alternative because many fringe disciplines have been in evidence for hundreds or, as in the case of reflexology, thousands of years, whereas Western medicine has been around only for about three hundred years, and modern drug-centred medicine only for about forty-five years. In terms of historical perspective, therefore, if nothing else, it seems unreasonable of the medical profession in general to be quite as dismissive as they sometimes are of some of the extraordinary ancient forms of healing.

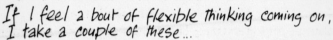

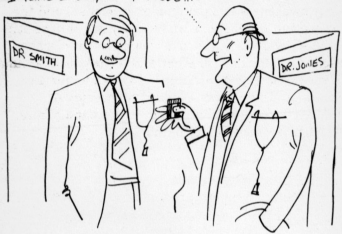

THE DIAGNOSTIC POWER OF REFLEXOLOGY

One of reflexology's greatest and most impressive strengths is its ability to make accurate diagnoses of conditions and symptoms. Often a patient will come in to a treatment session with a specific symptom in mind, but the reflexologist will, during the treatment, frequently be able to pick up on several other areas which might be out of balance. (Examples of this might be frustrations at work, loneliness, the feeling of something missing from your life, and an inability to express certain emotions or to 'speak your own mind'.) It is often found that the symptoms are linked, as explained in the description of the zone theory (page 7).

CONCLUSION

As has been pointed out throughout this book, patterns and connections can be seen at many levels. They can be seen within our bodies, as exemplified by the very nature of reflexology and the zone theory; they can be seen, too, within our beings in the interaction of the different levels of our selves – physical, mental, emotional and spiritual. The more we are able to open up our awareness to this complex interplay, and the more we can realize that we function not only as self-contained systems but also as complementary ones (complementary to each other and to the world around us), the more we will open up pathways to our true potential and happiness. And in the healing of ourselves we will be able also to understand others more clearly, and heal them too.

FURTHER READING

Bayly, Doreen E., *Reflexology Today*, Thorsons, 1982.

Byers, Dwight C., *Better Health with Foot Reflexology*, Ingham Publishing, 1983.

Goosmann-Legger, Astrid I., *Zone Therapy Using Foot Massage*, C.W. Daniel 1986.

Hall, Nicola M., *Reflexology – a Patient's Guide*, Thorsons, 1986.

Hall, Nicola M., *Reflexology – A Way to Better Health*, Pan, 1988.

Ingham Stopfel, Eunice, *Stories the Feet Can Tell*, Ingham Publishing, 1959.

Ingham Stopfel, Eunice, *Stories the Feet Have Told*, Ingham Publishing, 1959.

Kaye, Anna and Matchan, Don C., *Reflexology – Techniques of Foot Massage for Health and Fitness*, Thorsons, 1979.

Marquardt, Hanne, *Reflex Zone Therapy of the Feet*, Thorsons, 1983.

USEFUL ADDRESSES

For information on where to find a good practitioner, the following addresses will be useful.

UK

Association of Reflexologists
Slaters
Willow End
London
N20 8EP

and

Hodgson's Cottage
51 West End Lane
Esher
Surrey
KT10 8LF

The Bayly School of Reflexology
Monks Orchard
Whitbourne
Worcester
WR6 5RB

USA

New York School for Shiatsu and Reflexology
149 East 81st Street
New York City
NY 10028

Reflexology/Ministry of Healing
3828 Kramer Street
Harrisburg
PA 17109

Reflexology Workshop
1533 Shattuck
Berkeley
CA 94709

Europe

L'ASER (L'Association Suisse pour l'Etude de la
Reflexologie)
214 route des Convers
2616 Renan
Switzerland

CIRF (Centro Italiano Riflessologia Fitzgerald)
Via Bronzino 11
20133 Milan
Italy

INDEX

Numbers in *italic* refer to illustrations

MORE BOOKS FROM OPTIMA

ALTERNATIVE HEALTH SERIES

This series is designed to provide factual information and practical advice about alternative therapies. While including essential details of theory and history, the books concentrate on what patients can expect during treatment, how they should prepare for it, what questions will be asked and why, what form the treatment will take, and what it will 'feel' like and how soon they can expect to respond.

ACUPUNCTURE by Dr Michael Nightingale
Acupuncture is a traditional Chinese therapy which usually (but not always) uses needles to stimulate the body's own energy and so bring healing.
ISBN 0 356 12426 6
Price (in UK only) **£3.95**

ALEXANDER TECHNIQUE by Chris Stevens
Alexander Technique is a way of becoming more aware of balance, posture and movement in everyday activities. It can not only cure various complaints related to posture, such as backache, but teaches people to use their body more effectively and reduces stress.
ISBN 0 356 12430 4
Price (in UK only) **£4.99**

AROMATHERAPY by Gill Martin
Aromatherapy uses the essential oils of plants, which are massaged into the skin, added to baths or taken internally to treat a variety of ailments and enhance general well-being.
ISBN 0 356 17113 2
Price (in UK only) **£4.99**

CHIROPRACTIC by Susan Moore
Chiropractic is based on the belief that disease is
caused by the misalignment of the bones in the spine.
Chiropractors heal by manipulating the spine gently
back into its correct position.
ISBN 0 356 12433 9
Price (in UK only) **£3.95**

HERBAL MEDICINE by Anne McIntyre
Herbal medicine has been known for thousands of
years. It is an entirely natural system of medicine
which relies on the therapeutic quality of plants to
enhance the body's recuperative powers, and so bring
health – without any undesirable side effects.
ISBN 0 356 12429 0
Price (in UK only) **£3.95**

HOMEOPATHY by Dr Nelson Brunton
Homeopathy is based on the principle, discovered by
Samuel Hahnemann some 200 years ago, that like
cures like. In this system of medicine, diseases are
treated with very small quantities of herbs, minerals or
drugs.
ISBN 0 356 12427 4
Price (in UK only) **£4.99**

HYPNOSIS by Ursula Markham
Hypnosis has a remarkable record of curing a wide
range of ills. Ursula Markham a practising
hypnotherapist, explains how, by releasing inner
tensions, hypnosis can help people to heal themselves.
ISBN 0 356 12432 0
Price (in UK only) **£3.95**

MEDITATION by Erica Smith and Nicholas Wilks
Meditation is a state of inner stillness which has been
cultivated by mystics for thousands of years. The main
reason for its recent popularity is that regular practice
has been found to improve mental and physical health,
largely due to its role in alleviating stress.
ISBN 0 356 14569 7
Price (in UK only) **£4.99**

OSTEOPATHY by Stephen Sandler
Osteopathy started in the USA in the 1870s, and has since spread to many other countries. It is a manipulative therapy, in which the osteopath heals by adjusting the position of bones and tissues.
ISBN 0 356 12428 2
Price (in UK only) **£3.95**

All Optima books are available at your bookshop or newsagent, or can be ordered from the following address:

Optima, Cash Sales Department,
PO Box 11, Falmouth, Cornwall TR10 9EN

Please send cheque or postal order (no currency), and allow 60p for postage and packing for the first book, plus 25p for the second book and 15p for each additional book ordered up to a maximum charge of £1.90 in the UK.

Customers in Eire and BFPO please allow 60p for the first book, 25p for the second book plus 15p per copy for the next 7 books, thereafter 9p per book.

Overseas customers please allow £1.25 for postage and packing for the first book and 28p per copy for each additional book.

ANYA GORE is a practising reflexologist and masseuse. She can be contacted for advice and treatment through the publishers.